ARIA EVERGREEN

EmpowerFit 30-Day Fitness Challenge for Women

Contents

Preface

Designed to uplift both mind and body, this empowering journey encompasses dynamic Fusion Workouts, balanced nutrition, and self-care practices. At the end of the book, you'll find a day-by-day challenge cheat sheet—a comprehensive guide offering empowering sample workouts for each day of the 30-day challenge. Whether you choose to follow this cheat sheet or customize your EmpowerFit experience, these workouts will propel you toward strength and grace, guiding you to thrive in your unique journey. So, seize this opportunity to ignite your inner fire, rise strong, and embark on a life filled with vitality and confidence. EmpowerFit awaits, and the choice to embrace your empowerment is yours.

As you embark on this empowering journey with EmpowerFit, I want to extend my heartfelt gratitude for choosing to be a part of this empowering community. Your commitment to personal growth and well-being means the world to me, and I truly hope that this book serves as a guiding light on your path to empowerment.

If you find value, inspiration, and empowerment within the pages of EmpowerFit, I kindly ask you to take a moment to leave a review on Amazon or any other platform where you purchased this book. Your honest feedback will not only help others discover the transformative power of EmpowerFit, but it will also enable me to continue creating empowering content for women like you.

Your voice matters, and your review can inspire and empower countless other women to rise strong and embrace their own unique journeys. Thank you for being an integral part of the EmpowerFit community, and together, let's spread the spirit of empowerment far and wide.

Introduction

Welcome to EmpowerFit

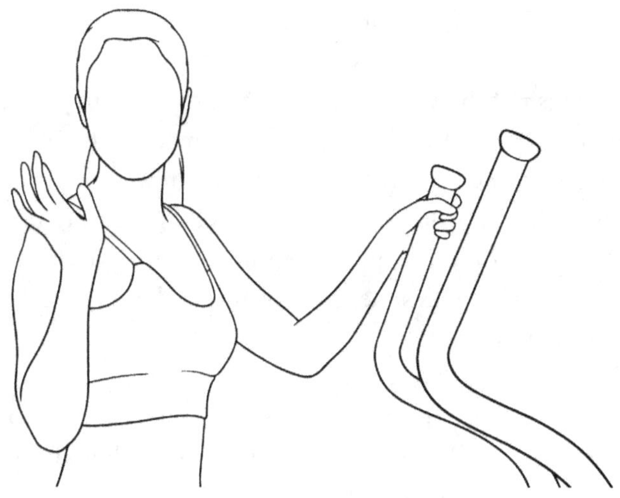

Dear Readers, Welcome to "EmpowerFit: 30-Day Fitness Challenge for Women"! We are thrilled to embark on this transformative journey with you, as we take a step towards empowering ourselves both physically and mentally.

In a world that often demands so much from us, we may find ourselves neglecting the most crucial aspect of our lives—our well-being. This book was created with a single purpose in mind: to help you reclaim that lost connection with yourself, discover your inner strength, and embrace a healthier and more confident version of YOU.

The EmpowerFit 30-Day Fitness Challenge is more than just a series of workouts; it's a holistic approach to self-improvement. Through carefully crafted exercises, nourishing nutrition guidance, and empowering mindset tips, we aim to support you in achieving your fitness goals while nurturing a positive body image and mental well-being.

Our goal is not to promote unrealistic expectations or drastic transformations. Instead, we want to encourage you to set personalized and achievable goals that align with your unique journey. Whether you're a fitness enthusiast looking to reignite your passion or a complete beginner taking the first step towards an active lifestyle, EmpowerFit is here to guide you every step of the way.

Throughout these 30 days, you'll challenge yourself, break barriers, and celebrate your successes—both big and small. This challenge is about embracing progress over perfection, recognizing that every step forward is a triumph in itself.

Within these pages, you'll find a carefully structured program designed to progressively build your strength, endurance, and flexibility. We'll incorporate diverse workouts, including cardio, strength training, yoga, and pilates, ensuring a well-rounded and engaging experience.

Moreover, we understand that fitness is not solely about physical prowess; it's a journey that encompasses the mind as well. You'll discover the power of self-care, mindfulness, and positive affirmations to cultivate a healthy relationship with yourself. EmpowerFit is not just about sculpting your body; it's about nurturing your soul.

As you embrace the challenge, remember that you are not alone on this path. Together, we'll form a supportive community of women uplifting one another, celebrating each other's achievements, and providing encouragement during moments of doubt.

At the end of these 30 days, you will emerge stronger, more resilient, and filled with an immense sense of accomplishment. This is your journey—your opportunity to break free from self-doubt and embrace your true potential.

Are you ready to embark on this empowering adventure? We believe in you, and we are honored to be your companions on this quest for growth and self-discovery.

Let's begin the EmpowerFit 30-Day Fitness Challenge and

create a life-changing story, one day at a time!

With love and support,

Aria Evergreen

The EmpowerFit Journey

Embracing Strength and Confidence

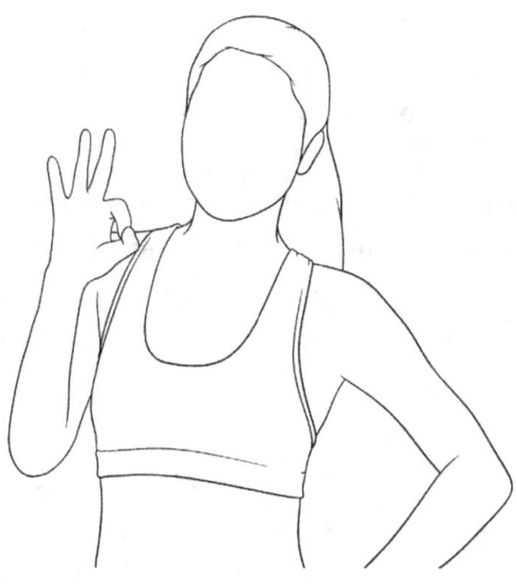

Setting realistic fitness goals and managing expectations during the 30-day challenge is of utmost significance as it forms the foundation for a successful and sustainable fitness journey. It is natural to be enthusiastic and motivated when starting a new challenge, but unrealistic goals or expectations can lead to frustration, burnout, and a higher likelihood of giving up prematurely.

1. Sustainable Progress: When it comes to getting fit, it's super important to set achievable goals. That way, you can work towards them at a steady pace and make progress that you can maintain in the long run. Instead of trying to make huge changes all at once, focus on making small improvements that you can stick to even after your fitness challenge is over. Trust me, it'll be much easier and more rewarding in the end!

2. Boosting Motivation: Staying motivated for the 30-day challenge becomes easier when you set achievable goals. Small successes along the way give you a feeling of accomplishment, which helps you stay determined to keep moving forward.

3. Preventing Overexertion and Injuries: Unrealistic expectations might push you to overexert yourself, leading to injuries or burnout. By setting achievable goals, you can design a workout plan that challenges you without risking your well-being.

4. Building Confidence: Meeting realistic fitness goals cultivates a sense of confidence in your abilities. Each milestone reached reinforces your belief in yourself, encouraging you to keep striving for further achievements.

5. Adapting to Individual Needs: Recognize that everyone's fitness journey is unique. Setting realistic goals allows you to tailor the challenge to your specific needs and fitness level, ensuring that you remain engaged and committed.

6. Focusing on Personal Growth: The 30-day challenge is an opportunity for personal growth, both physically and mentally. By managing expectations, you can shift the focus from external comparisons to your own progress, making the journey more fulfilling.

7. Embracing a Positive Mindset: Unrealistic goals can lead to self-criticism and negative self-talk when you perceive yourself falling short. By setting attainable objectives, you can foster a positive mindset, celebrating every step forward and learning from setbacks.

8. Long-Term Lifestyle Change: The purpose of the EmpowerFit 30-Day Fitness Challenge is not just a temporary transformation but a lasting lifestyle change. Realistic goals help you develop habits that can be sustained beyond the challenge, promoting continued growth and well-being.

9. Enjoying the Journey: Fitness is not solely about the destination but the journey itself. Setting realistic goals allows you to enjoy the process, finding joy in the workouts, nourishing meals, and self-improvement along the way.

10. Inspiring Others: As you achieve your realistic fitness goals, you become an inspiration to others in the community. Your progress motivates and encourages fellow participants to keep pushing forward, creating a supportive and uplifting environment.

Remember, the EmpowerFit challenge is about embracing progress, not perfection. Be kind to yourself, celebrate your achievements, and recognize that each step forward, no matter how small, is a remarkable accomplishment. Together, let's make the most of this empowering 30-day journey and embrace the beauty of growth and self-discovery.

Setting the Foundation

Assessing Your Fitness and Well-Being

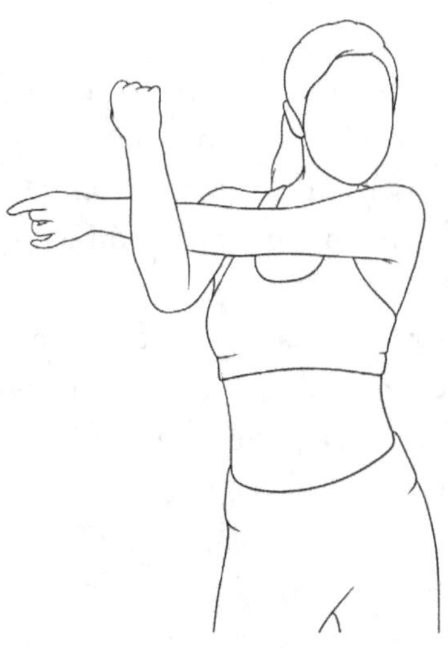

The importance of self-care and health in women's lives cannot be overstated, as it forms the foundation for overall well-being and a fulfilling life. Prioritizing self-care is not a luxury but a necessity for maintaining physical, mental, and emotional health. Here are some key reasons why women should prioritize their well-being:

1. **Physical Health:** Taking care of one's body is vital for optimal physical health. Regular exercise, nutritious eating habits, and sufficient rest help in preventing chronic diseases, improving cardiovascular health, and boosting the immune system.

2. **Mental Well-Being:** Self-care is essential for maintaining mental and emotional health. Engaging in activities that promote relaxation, stress reduction, and mindfulness can help alleviate anxiety, depression, and burnout.

3. **Increased Resilience:** When women prioritize their well-being, they build resilience to cope with life's challenges. Self-care equips them with the mental and emotional strength to face adversity and bounce back from difficult situations.

4. **Enhanced Productivity:** Taking time for self-care can improve productivity. When women feel physically and mentally energized, they can perform better in their personal and professional lives.

5. **Positive Body Image:** Self-care encourages women to appreciate and love their bodies, regardless of societal expectations. By valuing their health over unrealistic beauty standards,

women can develop a positive body image and higher self-esteem.

6. Stress Reduction: Women often face multiple responsibilities and roles, leading to stress and overwhelm. Prioritizing self-care provides a much-needed break, reducing stress levels and promoting a sense of calm.

7. Improved Relationships: When women take care of themselves, they are better able to nurture healthy relationships with others. Prioritizing well-being enables them to show up as their best selves in personal connections.

8. Setting a Positive Example: Prioritizing self-care sets a positive example for younger generations, encouraging them to value their well-being and make self-care a priority in their lives.

9. Life Balance: Self-care helps women strike a balance between work, family, and personal interests. By taking time for themselves, they avoid burnout and maintain a fulfilling lifestyle.

10. Long-Term Health: Investing in self-care today ensures better long-term health outcomes. It reduces the risk of chronic illnesses and supports healthy aging, allowing women to lead active and vibrant lives as they grow older.

11. Empowerment and Independence: Prioritizing self-care empowers women to take charge of their health and well-being. It fosters a sense of independence and self-reliance.

12. Happiness and Fulfillment: Self-care contributes to overall happiness and life satisfaction. When women prioritize their well-being, they experience a sense of fulfillment and contentment in their lives.

Fueling Your Empowerment

Nutrition and Hydration Essentials

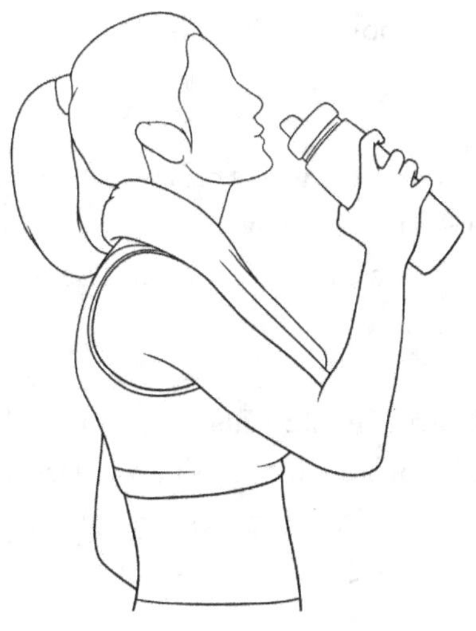

Proper nutrition and hydration play a vital role in achieving fitness goals as they directly impact the body's ability to perform, recover, and adapt to exercise. Without adequate nourishment and hydration, even the most well-designed workout plan may fall short of yielding desired results. Here are the basics of proper nutrition and hydration and their significance in reaching fitness goals:

1. Fueling the Body: Nutrition provides the essential nutrients needed to fuel the body for physical activity. Carbohydrates are the primary source of energy, while proteins aid in muscle repair and growth. Fats also play a crucial role in supporting sustained energy during longer workouts.

2. Supporting Exercise Performance: Proper nutrition ensures that the body has the energy reserves to perform at its best during workouts. Well-balanced meals with a mix of macronutrients optimize stamina and prevent premature fatigue.

3. Muscle Recovery and Repair: After exercise, muscles need proper nutrients to recover and repair. Adequate protein intake supports muscle tissue repair and helps prevent muscle soreness and injuries.

4. Building Lean Muscle Mass: For individuals aiming to build lean muscle, protein intake is particularly crucial. Protein provides the building blocks necessary for muscle growth and helps preserve existing muscle mass during weight loss.

5. Enhancing Endurance: Proper nutrition ensures that the body has enough glycogen (stored carbohydrates) to sustain endurance activities. This is especially important for endurance athletes or those participating in longer workouts.

6. Hydration for Optimal Performance: Hydration is key for regulating body temperature and preventing dehydration during physical activity. Even mild dehydration can negatively impact exercise performance and cognitive function.

7. Electrolyte Balance: Sweating during exercise leads to the loss of electrolytes, such as sodium, potassium, and magnesium. Proper hydration with electrolyte-rich fluids helps maintain the body's balance and prevents cramps and muscle weakness.

8. Metabolism and Weight Management: Proper nutrition supports a healthy metabolism, which is essential for weight management and body composition goals. Balanced meals with appropriate portion sizes aid in weight loss or maintenance.

9. Immune System Support: Proper nutrition helps bolster the immune system, reducing the risk of illnesses that could interfere with consistent workouts.

10. Recovery and Adaptation: After exercise, nutrition plays a crucial role in the body's recovery and adaptation processes. Nutrients from food support muscle repair and replenish glycogen stores, preparing the body for subsequent workouts.

11. Mental Focus and Clarity: Good nutrition supports mental clarity and focus, contributing to better exercise performance and adherence to workout plans.

By understanding the importance of proper nutrition and hydration, individuals can make informed choices about their dietary habits and optimize their fitness journey. EmpowerFit emphasizes the significance of balanced and nourishing meals, as well as the value of staying hydrated to empower women in achieving their fitness goals and leading healthier, more fulfilling lives.

Week 1: Building Strength and Resilience

Foundation-Building Exercises

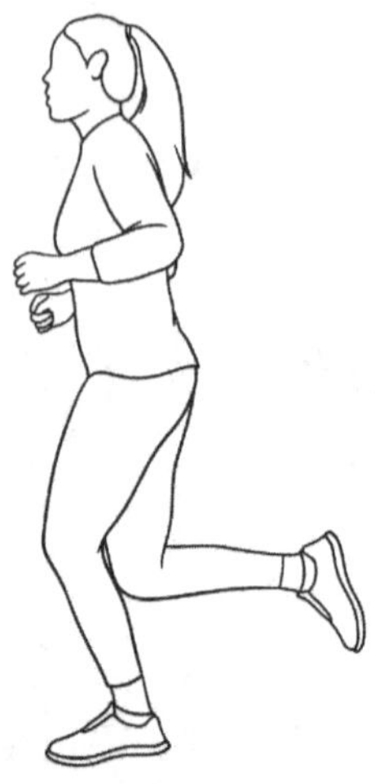

Week 1: Foundation-Building

In Week 1 of the EmpowerFit 30-Day Fitness Challenge, we focus on laying the foundation for your fitness journey. These foundation-building exercises aim to improve flexibility, enhance cardiovascular endurance, and introduce you to basic strength training movements. The week starts with a gentle warm-up and stretching routine to prepare your body for the upcoming workouts.

Day 1:

1. Warm-up (5 minutes):

- Start with light cardio, such as brisk walking or jogging in place, to raise your heart rate.

- Perform arm circles, leg swings, and hip rotations to warm up the major joints.

2. Stretching (7 minutes):
   - Hold each stretch for 20-30 seconds:
   - Neck stretch
   - Shoulder stretch
   - Triceps stretch
   - Quad stretch
   - Hamstring stretch
   - Calf stretch

3. Foundation Exercise - Cardiovascular Endurance:
   - Choose your preferred cardio activity: brisk walking, jogging, cycling, or dancing.
   - Perform 20-30 minutes of continuous activity, aiming to keep your heart rate elevated.

Day 2:
   1. Warm-up (5 minutes):
   - Repeat the warm-up routine from Day 1 to gradually increase your body's temperature.

2. Stretching (7 minutes):
   - Repeat the stretching routine from Day 1, focusing on maintaining proper form and deepening the stretches.

3. Foundation Exercise - Strength Training (Upper Body):
   - Perform bodyweight exercises such as push-ups, modified push-ups, and triceps dips.
   - Aim for 3 sets of 10-12 repetitions for each exercise, with short rests between sets.

Day 3:

1. Warm-up (5 minutes):
- Repeat the warm-up routine from Day 1.

2. Stretching (7 minutes):
- Repeat the stretching routine from Day 1, focusing on relaxing and breathing deeply during the stretches.

3. Foundation Exercise - Strength Training (Lower Body):
- Perform bodyweight squats, lunges, and glute bridges.
- Aim for 3 sets of 10-12 repetitions for each exercise, with short rests between sets.

Day 4:
1. Rest Day:
- Take a day off from structured workouts to allow your body to recover and repair.

Day 5:
1. Warm-up (5 minutes):
- Repeat the warm-up routine from Day 1.

2. Stretching (7 minutes):
- Repeat the stretching routine from Day 1, focusing on increasing flexibility and range of motion.

3. Foundation Exercise - Full-Body Circuit:
- Create a circuit combining bodyweight exercises for the upper and lower body, along with a brief burst of cardiovascular exercise (e.g., jumping jacks).
- Perform each exercise for 30 seconds, then move to the next exercise without rest.

- Complete 3 rounds of the circuit, resting for 1 minute between rounds.

Day 6:
  1. Warm-up (5 minutes):
  - Repeat the warm-up routine from Day 1.

2. Stretching (7 minutes):
  - Repeat the stretching routine from Day 1, focusing on maintaining proper alignment and balance.

3. Foundation Exercise - Flexibility:
  - Practice a gentle yoga or Pilates session to improve flexibility and promote relaxation.

Day 7:
  1. Rest Day:
  - Enjoy a rest day to give your body time to recover and rejuvenate.

Throughout Week 1, remember to stay hydrated and listen to your body. The foundation exercises will prepare you for more challenging workouts in the upcoming weeks. Each day, take a moment to reflect on your progress and celebrate the commitment you've made to your fitness journey. As you embrace these foundational exercises, know that you are already on the path to empowerment and strength!

Cardiovascular Endurance Workouts

In Week 1 of the EmpowerFit 30-Day Fitness Challenge, readers can incorporate various cardiovascular endurance workouts to improve their cardiovascular fitness and stamina. These exercises are beginner-friendly and can be modified based on individual fitness levels. The goal is to engage in activities that elevate the heart rate and keep it elevated for an extended period. Here are some cardiovascular endurance workouts for Week 1:

Day 1:

  - **Brisk Walking:** Start with a 20-30 minute brisk walk in your neighborhood or a nearby park. Maintain a pace that elevates your heart rate but allows you to carry on a conversation.

Day 3:

  - **Jogging or Running:** If you're comfortable with jogging or running, go for a 15-20 minute jog or run. If you're a beginner, you can try a walk-jog interval, alternating between walking and jogging for 1-2 minutes each.

Day 5:

  - **Cycling:** Hop on a stationary bike or go for a leisurely bike ride outdoors for 20-30 minutes. Adjust the resistance or terrain to challenge yourself.

Day 7:

  - **Jumping Rope:** Grab a skipping rope and perform a 10-15 minute jump rope session. Start with single jumps and progress to double unders as you become more proficient.

Throughout Week 1:
   - **Dance Cardio:** Incorporate 10-15 minutes of dance cardio into your daily routine. Put on your favorite music and dance freely, enjoying the rhythm and movement.

- **Stair Climbing:** If you have access to stairs, include a 10-15 minute stair-climbing session. Climb up and down the stairs, focusing on proper form and balance.

- **High-Intensity Interval Training (HIIT):** Try a beginner-friendly HIIT workout, consisting of short bursts of intense exercise (e.g., jumping jacks, high knees, or burpees) followed by brief periods of rest or low-intensity activity.

Remember to start at a pace that suits your fitness level and gradually increase the intensity and duration of the workouts as you progress. Stay hydrated throughout each session and listen to your body's cues. Cardiovascular endurance workouts not only improve your heart health but also boost your mood and energy levels. Have fun exploring different activities and find what brings you joy and excitement during your Week 1 fitness journey!

Strength Training for Beginners

During Week 1 of the EmpowerFit 30-Day Fitness Challenge, we will introduce beginners to fundamental strength training exercises that lay the groundwork for building muscle and increasing overall strength. Strength training is essential for women as it promotes bone health, boosts metabolism, and enhances functional fitness. Here are some beginner-friendly strength training exercises with explanations of proper form and technique:

1. Bodyweight Squats:
   - Stand with feet hip-width apart, toes slightly turned out.
   - Keep your chest lifted, core engaged, and shoulders relaxed.
   - Lower your hips back and down as if sitting in a chair, ensuring your knees track over your toes.
   - Aim for thighs parallel to the ground or slightly below.
   - Push through your heels to return to the starting position.

2. Push-Ups:
   - Start in a plank position with hands placed slightly wider than shoulder-width apart.
   - Lower your body towards the floor, keeping your elbows close to your sides.
   - Lower until your chest is just above the ground, then push back up to the plank position.
   - Modify by doing push-ups on your knees or against a wall if the standard push-up is challenging.

3. Glute Bridges:
   - Lie on your back with knees bent and feet flat on the floor, hip-width apart.
   - Engage your glutes and core as you lift your hips off the ground, forming a straight line from shoulders to knees.
   - Squeeze your glutes at the top, then lower your hips back

to the floor.

4. Modified Plank:

- Start on your hands and knees, with wrists directly under your shoulders and knees under your hips.
- Extend your legs back, keeping your body in a straight line from head to heels.
- Engage your core and hold this position, avoiding arching or rounding your back.

5. Dumbbell Bicep Curls:

- Stand with feet shoulder-width apart, holding a dumbbell in each hand with palms facing forward.
- Keep your elbows close to your sides and curl the dumbbells towards your shoulders.
- Lower the weights back down in a controlled manner.

6. Dumbbell Bent-Over Rows:

- Stand with feet hip-width apart, holding a dumbbell in each hand with palms facing your body.
- Hinge at the hips to bend forward slightly, keeping your back flat and core engaged.
- Pull the dumbbells towards your ribcage, squeezing your shoulder blades together.
- Lower the weights back down with control.

Remember to start with lighter weights or no weights at all to focus on mastering proper form. Perform 2-3 sets of 10-12 repetitions for each exercise, with short rests in between sets. As a beginner, it's crucial to prioritize form over weight, ensuring your movements are safe and effective. Feel free to seek guidance from a fitness professional if you have any concerns about technique or if you need modifications to accommodate individual needs and abilities. Embrace these foundational strength training exercises, and you'll be on your way to developing a strong, empowered body during Week 1 and beyond!

Staying Driven and Inspired

Staying committed and driven throughout the 30-day challenge is essential for achieving your fitness goals and embracing the EmpowerFit journey to its fullest. Here are some motivational tips to keep you focused and inspired throughout the challenge:

1. Set Clear and Attainable Goals: Define specific, measurable, and realistic fitness goals for the 30-day challenge. Break them down into smaller milestones to track your progress and celebrate your achievements along the way.

2. Visualize Success: Create a mental image of yourself accomplishing your fitness goals. Visualization can boost confidence and motivation, making it easier to stay committed to the challenge.

3. Create a Supportive Environment: Surround yourself with positive and like-minded individuals who encourage and uplift you. Join fitness communities, share your progress, and seek inspiration from others' journeys.

4. Keep a Workout Journal: Maintain a workout journal to track your daily exercise, nutrition, and thoughts. Reviewing your progress can help you stay accountable and motivated to continue pushing forward.

5. Celebrate Small Wins: Celebrate each accomplishment, no matter how small. Recognize your efforts and reward yourself with non-food treats to reinforce positive behaviors.

6. Embrace Progress Over Perfection: Acknowledge that progress is not always linear, and setbacks are a natural part of the journey. Focus on continuous improvement and learning from challenges.

7. Positive Self-Talk: Replace self-doubt with positive affirmations. Remind yourself of your strengths and capabilities, affirming that you are capable of conquering any obstacles.

8. Find Joy in Movement: Discover physical activities you genuinely enjoy. Whether it's dancing, hiking, or playing a sport, finding pleasure in movement makes workouts more fulfilling.

9. Remind Yourself of the "Why": Reconnect with your reasons for starting the challenge. Whether it's improving your health, building confidence, or setting an example for loved ones, keeping the "why" in mind fuels your dedication.

10. Be Flexible and Adaptable: Embrace the ebb and flow of life, and be flexible with your workout routine. If you miss a day or need to adjust your plan, don't be discouraged—start again the next day.

11. Visual Progress Tracking: Take progress photos or measurements to observe physical changes over time. Seeing tangible results can be highly motivating.

12. Motivational Quotes and Affirmations: Surround yourself with motivational quotes and affirmations that resonate with your goals. Place them where you can see them daily for a boost of inspiration.

13. Treat Yourself with Kindness: Be gentle with yourself and avoid self-criticism. Celebrate the effort you put into each workout and recognize that consistency is key to success.

14. Remain Curious and Open-Minded: Stay curious about your body and its capabilities. Embrace new exercises and challenges with an open mind, discovering what works best for you.

15. Focus on the Journey, Not the Destination: Remember that the EmpowerFit challenge is about personal growth and self-improvement. Enjoy the process, and let the journey unfold with each day.

By incorporating these motivational tips into your daily routine, you can stay committed and driven throughout the 30-day challenge. Your dedication and determination will empower you to overcome obstacles and achieve the transformation you seek—both physically and mentally. Keep pushing forward, and remember that you have the strength and resilience to make this journey a remarkable success!

Week 2: Empowering with Cardio and Strength

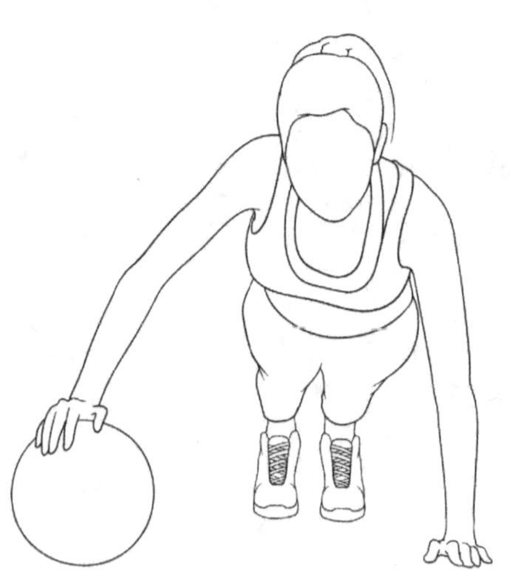

Welcome to Week 2 of the EmpowerFit 30-Day Fitness Challenge! In Week 2, we shift our focus to strength and toning exercises, incorporating resistance training to elevate your fitness journey to new heights. Resistance training, also known as strength training or weight training, involves using external resistance to challenge your muscles. This type of exercise is crucial for women's fitness for several reasons:

1. Building Lean Muscle Mass: Resistance training stimulates muscle growth and development, helping you build lean muscle mass. Increased muscle mass not only enhances your strength but also boosts your metabolism, making it easier to manage body composition and weight.

2. Toning and Definition: Incorporating resistance exercises helps tone and define your muscles, giving your body a sculpted and athletic appearance.

3. Strengthening Bones: Resistance training is beneficial for bone health, reducing the risk of osteoporosis and promoting bone density.

4. Improving Functional Fitness: Strength training enhances your functional fitness, making everyday tasks easier to perform. This includes activities like carrying groceries, lifting objects, and maintaining balance.

5. Increasing Strength and Power: As you progressively challenge your muscles with resistance, you'll notice an improvement in overall strength and power. This can translate into better athletic performance and increased endurance.

6. Injury Prevention: Strengthening your muscles and connective tissues through resistance training can help prevent injuries during physical activities and sports.

7. Enhancing Metabolism: Muscle is metabolically active tissue, meaning it burns more calories at rest compared to fat. As you increase your muscle mass through resistance training, your resting metabolic rate improves, supporting weight management and overall health.

Now, let's dive into some strength and toning exercises that you can incorporate into Week 2:

1. Dumbbell Squats: Hold a dumbbell in each hand at shoulder height, and perform squats with proper form as you did in Week 1.

2. Dumbbell Lunges: Hold dumbbells in each hand and step forward into lunges, alternating legs. Keep your back straight and chest lifted throughout the movement.

3. Dumbbell Shoulder Press: Stand tall with dumbbells at shoulder level. Press them overhead, fully extending your arms, and lower them back down.

4. Dumbbell Rows: Bend forward with a slight bend in your knees, holding dumbbells in each hand. Pull the dumbbells towards your ribcage, squeezing your shoulder blades together, and then lower them down.

5. Plank with Shoulder Taps: From a plank position, lift one hand to tap the opposite shoulder while maintaining a stable core and neutral spine. Alternate sides.

6. Tricep Dips: Use a stable surface, such as a chair or bench. Place your hands on the edge, fingers pointing forward, and lower your body down by bending your elbows. Push back up to the starting position.

As you progress through Week 2, remember to choose dumbbell weights that challenge you without compromising proper form. Perform 2-3 sets of 10-12 repetitions for each exercise, with short rests in between sets. Combine these strength and toning exercises with your cardiovascular workouts from Week 1 for a well-rounded fitness routine that empowers you to reach new levels of strength and confidence. Keep pushing forward, and let Week 2 become a stepping stone to even greater achievements in the weeks ahead!

Cardiovascular and Strength Workouts Combined

Combining cardio and strength workouts is a powerful approach that enhances overall fitness levels and offers a host of benefits for women on their fitness journey. This synergy between cardiovascular exercise and strength training creates a balanced and comprehensive fitness routine that maximizes results. Here are the key benefits of combining cardio and strength workouts:

1. **Improved Cardiovascular Health:** Cardiovascular exercises, such as running, cycling, and dancing, elevate the heart rate and improve cardiovascular endurance. This type of exercise strengthens the heart and lungs, promoting better circulation and oxygen delivery throughout the body.

2. **Increased Muscle Strength and Tone:** Strength training exercises challenge the muscles, leading to increased strength and tone. Combining these exercises with cardio helps target various muscle groups, creating a balanced and well-rounded physique.

3. **Enhanced Caloric Burn:** Cardio workouts are effective for burning calories during the activity itself. However, strength training also contributes to post-workout calorie burn. As muscles repair and rebuild after strength workouts, the body expends energy, leading to an increase in overall calorie expenditure.

4. **Boosted Metabolism:** The combination of cardio and strength workouts can lead to an increased resting metabolic rate. As lean muscle mass grows from strength training, the body burns more calories even at rest, supporting weight management and body composition goals.

5. **Optimized Fat Loss:** The synergy of cardio and strength exercises is excellent for fat loss. Cardio workouts help burn stored fat, while strength training preserves muscle mass during weight loss, preventing muscle loss commonly associated with calorie restriction.

6. Improved Endurance: Cardiovascular workouts improve endurance, allowing you to sustain physical activity for longer periods. This increased stamina enhances performance during strength training and everyday activities.

7. Better Bone Health: Both cardio and strength exercises contribute to bone health. Cardio activities like jogging or dancing are weight-bearing exercises that strengthen bones, while resistance training supports bone density.

8. Reduced Risk of Chronic Diseases: Regularly combining cardio and strength workouts is associated with a reduced risk of chronic diseases, including cardiovascular disease, diabetes, and certain types of cancer.

9. Enhanced Functional Fitness: The combination of cardio and strength training improves functional fitness, making everyday tasks easier to perform and reducing the risk of injuries.

10. Mental Health Benefits: Cardio workouts release endorphins, improving mood and reducing stress. Strength training also has positive effects on mental well-being, boosting self-confidence and body image.

11. Versatility and Variety: Combining cardio and strength exercises allows for a wide range of workout options, preventing monotony and keeping your fitness routine fresh and exciting.

By integrating cardio and strength workouts into your fitness routine, you create a synergistic effect that maximizes the benefits of both types of exercise. The combination of improved cardiovascular health, increased muscle strength, optimized fat loss, and better overall fitness levels empowers you to achieve your fitness goals and lead a healthier, more vibrant life. The EmpowerFit challenge encourages the integration of cardio and strength workouts to support your journey toward strength, confidence, and well-being.

Embracing Progress

Moving Beyond Perfectionism

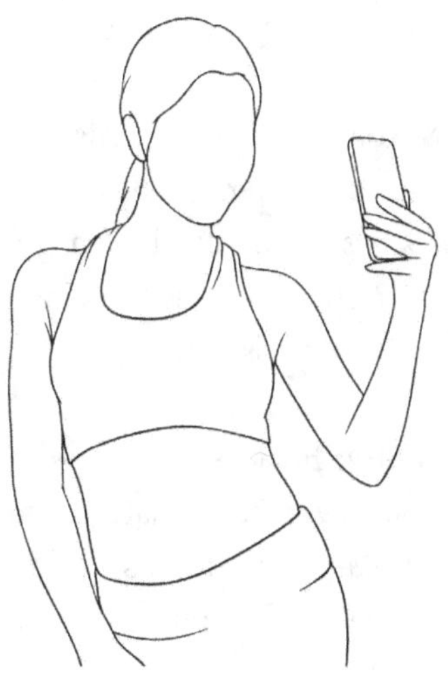

In your fitness journey, it's essential to acknowledge a common struggle that many of us face: the pursuit of perfection. As women striving for growth and empowerment, we often place immense pressure on ourselves to achieve flawless results in every aspect of life, including fitness. However, it's crucial to recognize that perfection is an unattainable standard, and the pursuit of it can be a hindrance rather than a motivator.

Embracing progress over perfection is the key to unlocking your true potential and enjoying the journey toward your goals. Here's why you should let go of perfectionism and celebrate every step of progress:

1. Celebrate Your Effort: Instead of focusing solely on the result, celebrate the effort you put into each workout and the dedication you show to your well-being. Every step you take, no matter how small, brings you closer to your aspirations.

2. Learn from Setbacks: Perfectionism can lead to fear of failure and avoidance of challenges. Embracing progress allows you to view setbacks as opportunities for growth and learning. When you encounter obstacles, see them as stepping stones to resilience and greater success.

3. Enjoy the Journey: Fitness is not solely about reaching a destination; it's about the transformation you experience along the way. Embrace the ups and downs, and find joy in the daily improvements you make. The journey itself is a beautiful and empowering experience.

4.   Personal Growth and Self-Discovery: Embracing progress encourages self-reflection and self-awareness. As you acknowledge your progress, you gain insight into your strengths, passions, and areas for growth, contributing to a deeper sense of self.

5. Set Realistic Goals: Perfectionism can lead to setting unattainable goals. Embracing progress allows you to set realistic, achievable targets, providing a sense of accomplishment and fueling your motivation to keep moving forward.

6. Build Resilience: Progress is not always linear, and that's okay. Embracing the journey strengthens your resilience, allowing you to bounce back from setbacks and stay committed to your fitness goals.

7. Celebrate Small Wins: Acknowledge and celebrate each small victory, as they accumulate significant achievements over time. Small wins are stepping stones to big accomplishments.

8. Practice Self-Compassion: Be kind to yourself when things don't go as planned. Treat yourself with the same compassion and encouragement you would offer a dear friend. Remember that you are worthy of love and acceptance, regardless of perceived imperfections.

9. Focus on Growth, Not Comparison: Progress is personal and unique to each individual. Avoid comparing yourself to others, as it undermines your journey. Instead, focus on your growth and what makes you feel strong and empowered.

10. Empower Yourself: Embracing progress empowers you to take ownership of your fitness journey and to define success on your terms. Trust in your ability to make positive changes and celebrate your achievements along the way.

Perfectionism may cast a shadow, but the light of progress shines bright. Embrace the beautiful journey you're embarking on, one step at a time. Each day, remind yourself that progress is a testament to your strength, determination, and growth. You are enough, just as you are, and your progress is a testament to your strength, determination, and growth. Trust in the process, and watch yourself bloom into a powerful, confident, and empowered woman. The EmpowerFit community stands with you, cheering you on every step of the way. Let progress be your guiding star as you shine brightly on this empowering 30-day journey and beyond.

Week 3: Finding Balance with Yoga and Pilates

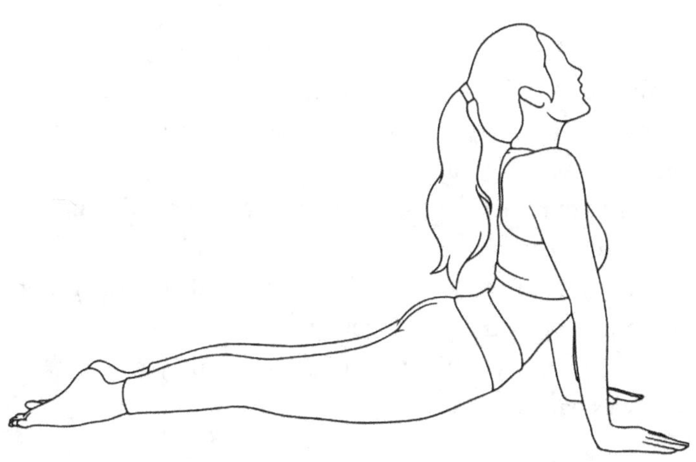

Welcome to Week 3 of the EmpowerFit 30-Day Fitness Challenge! This week, we'll incorporate yoga and Pilates exercises to enhance your flexibility, balance, and mind-body connection. These exercises focus on improving your range of motion, building core strength, and fostering a sense of inner peace. Let's dive into some yoga and Pilates exercises for Week 3:

1. Downward Dog (Adho Mukha Svanasana):

- Start on your hands and knees, aligning your wrists under your shoulders and knees under your hips.

- Tuck your toes, lift your hips, and straighten your legs, coming into an inverted V shape.

- Press your hands into the ground, lengthen your spine, and engage your core. Pedal your feet to stretch your calves and hamstrings.

2. Warrior II (Virabhadrasana II):

- From a standing position, step one foot back, keeping your feet about 3 to 4 feet apart.

- Turn your back foot slightly inward and bend your front knee over the ankle.

- Extend your arms out to the sides, parallel to the ground, and gaze over your front fingertips.

- This pose strengthens your legs, opens your hips, and improves balance.

3. Tree Pose (Vrksasana):

- Stand tall with feet hip-width apart. Shift your weight to one foot and lift the other foot off the ground.

- Place the sole of your lifted foot on the inner thigh of your standing leg or lower down on your calf, avoiding the knee.

- Bring your hands together in front of your heart or extend them overhead like branches.

- This pose challenges your balance and helps improve concentration.

4. Cat-Cow Stretch:

- Start on your hands and knees in a tabletop position.

- Inhale, arch your back and lift your head and tailbone towards the ceiling (Cow Pose).

- Exhale, round your back, and tuck your chin towards your chest (Cat Pose).

- Flow between these two positions, synchronizing movement with your breath.

5. Rolling Like a Ball:

- Sit on the floor with your knees bent, holding onto your shins.

- Balance on your sit bones as you tuck your chin and round your spine.

- Roll backward, then forward, using your core strength to maintain control.

6. Pilates Scissor Kick:

- Lie on your back, legs extended towards the ceiling.

- Lower one leg towards the floor as far as you can without arching your back, then switch legs in a scissor-like motion.

- This exercise strengthens your abdominal muscles and enhances lower body flexibility.

Remember to focus on your breath during these exercises,

allowing it to guide your movements and create a sense of relaxation. Yoga and Pilates provide a beautiful opportunity to connect with your body, embrace your strength, and find balance within yourself. Modify the poses as needed to suit your flexibility and comfort level. As you progress through Week 3, you'll notice improvements in your flexibility, balance, and overall sense of well-being. Embrace the grace and empowerment that yoga and Pilates bring to your fitness journey, and let Week 3 become a transformative experience on your path toward strength and self-discovery. Keep shining, EmpowerFit!

Enhancing Flexibility and Balance

Enhanced flexibility and balance offer a wealth of mental and physical benefits, making them valuable components of your fitness journey. As you incorporate yoga and Pilates exercises in Week 3 of the EmpowerFit challenge, you'll experience the positive impact these practices have on your overall well-being. Here are some of the mental and physical benefits of improved flexibility and balance:

Mental Benefits:

1. Stress Reduction: Flexibility-focused exercises, such as yoga, promote relaxation and activate the body's parasympathetic nervous system. This response helps reduce stress hormones like cortisol and induces a state of calmness, helping you manage stress more effectively.

2. Mindfulness and Presence: Flexibility and balance exercises encourage mindfulness—being fully present in the moment. Focusing on your breath and body movements during these exercises fosters mental clarity, allowing you to release distractions and cultivate a sense of centeredness.

3. Improved Concentration: Yoga and Pilates require mental focus and attention to alignment and breath. Practicing these exercises regularly can enhance your ability to concentrate and stay present in other areas of life.

4. Emotional Regulation: Enhanced flexibility and balance contribute to emotional well-being. The mind-body connection established through these practices can lead to improved emotional regulation and resilience in the face of challenges.

5. Enhanced Self-Awareness: Flexibility exercises encourage self-awareness, helping you become attuned to your body's sensations and limits. This heightened awareness extends beyond physical aspects to emotional and mental well-being, facilitating personal growth and self-discovery.

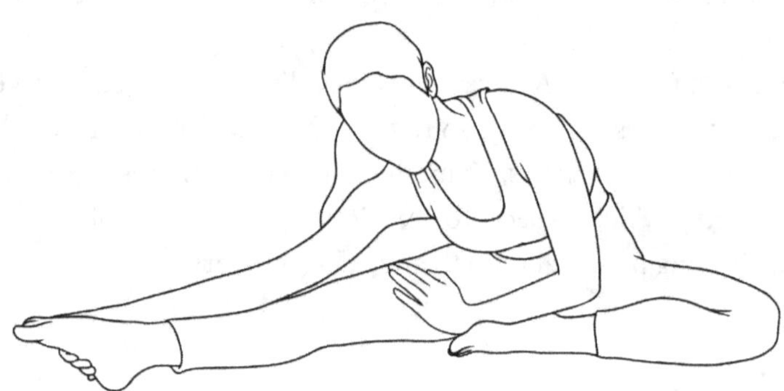

1. Improved Range of Motion: Enhanced flexibility allows joints to move more freely, improving the overall range of motion and reducing the risk of injuries related to muscle tightness or joint stiffness.

2. Increased Muscle Length: Regular stretching in yoga and Pilates elongates muscles, improving muscle flexibility and reducing muscle tension and soreness.

3. Better Posture: Improved flexibility and balance contribute to better alignment and posture. These exercises strengthen core muscles, which play a crucial role in supporting the spine and maintaining good posture.

4. Reduced Muscle Imbalances: Flexibility and balance exercises help address muscle imbalances that may occur due to repetitive movements or sedentary lifestyles, promoting optimal muscle function and reducing the risk of injury.

5. Joint Health: By improving flexibility and balance, you promote joint health and reduce the risk of joint-related issues, such as osteoarthritis.

6. Increased Circulation: Yoga and Pilates movements stimulate blood flow and enhance circulation, improving nutrient delivery to muscles and organs, which aids in their optimal functioning.

7. Muscle Recovery and Relaxation: Stretching and flexibility exercises promote muscle recovery, reducing muscle tension and promoting relaxation after intense workouts.

By embracing the mental and physical benefits of enhanced flexibility and balance, you cultivate a holistic approach to fitness and overall well-being. Yoga and Pilates offer you not only a stronger and more flexible body but also a calmer and more focused mind. Incorporating these practices into your fitness routine will empower you to move through life with grace, strength, and mindfulness. So, keep going, EmpowerFit, and let Week 3 be a transformative experience that nourishes both your body and soul!

Rest Days and Recovery

Nurturing Your Body and Mind

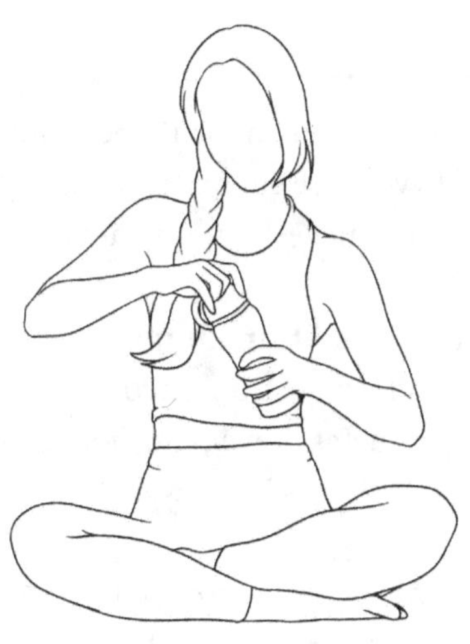

R est days and recovery are essential components of a well-rounded workout plan, and they play a crucial role in achieving optimal fitness and overall well-being. Here's why rest days are significant and some techniques for effective recovery:

Significance of Rest Days and Recovery:

1. Muscle Repair and Growth: During workouts, your muscles undergo micro-tears, and rest days provide the time needed for them to repair and rebuild. This repair process is crucial for muscle growth and strength development.

2. Injury Prevention: Rest days help prevent overuse injuries by allowing your body to recover from the stress and impact of intense workouts. Giving your muscles and joints time to recover reduces the risk of strains, sprains, and other injuries.

3. Enhanced Performance: Adequate rest and recovery enable your body to perform at its best during subsequent workouts. You'll have more energy, focus, and physical capacity to push harder and achieve greater results.

4. Reduced Fatigue and Burnout: Overtraining can lead to physical and mental exhaustion. Incorporating rest days and recovery techniques helps prevent burnout and maintains your enthusiasm for your fitness journey.

5. Hormonal Balance: Rest days help restore hormonal balance, including reducing cortisol levels (the stress hormone) and enhancing the production of growth hormones.

Techniques for Effective Recovery:

1. Active Recovery: Engage in low-intensity activities on rest days, such as walking, swimming, or gentle stretching. Active recovery promotes blood flow, which aids in the repair process while preventing stiffness.

2. Proper Nutrition: Eat a balanced diet that includes adequate protein to support muscle repair and carbohydrates to replenish glycogen stores. Hydrate well to assist in nutrient delivery and flush out toxins.

3. Sleep: Prioritize quality sleep, as it is crucial for physical and mental recovery. Aim for 7-9 hours of restful sleep each night to promote healing and muscle growth.

4. Foam Rolling and Self-Massage: Use foam rollers or massage tools to release muscle tension and knots. Self-massage helps improve circulation and reduce soreness.

5. Stretching and Flexibility Exercises: Incorporate regular stretching sessions to enhance flexibility, reduce muscle tightness, and improve overall range of motion.

6. Contrast Baths or Ice Baths: Alternating between hot and cold water immersion can help reduce inflammation and muscle soreness. Consult a healthcare professional if you have any medical conditions or concerns before trying this technique.

7. Meditation and Mindfulness: Practice relaxation techniques, such as meditation or deep breathing exercises, to reduce stress and promote mental recovery.

8. Listen to Your Body: Pay attention to how your body feels. If you experience persistent fatigue, soreness, or signs of overtraining, allow yourself additional rest and consider adjusting your workout plan.

9. Periodization: Incorporate periodization into your workout plan by alternating between high-intensity and lower-intensity training phases. This approach allows for proper recovery and prevents plateaus.

Remember that recovery is a vital part of progress, and it's okay to take rest days without guilt. Your body requires time to adapt and grow stronger. Embrace rest and recovery as an essential aspect of your fitness journey, and you'll find that it enhances your overall performance and empowers you to achieve your fitness goals with greater success and longevity. Keep nurturing yourself, EmpowerFit, and let Week 3 and beyond be filled with strength, flexibility, and balanced well-being!

Celebrating Self-Care

Nurturing Your Mind and Soul

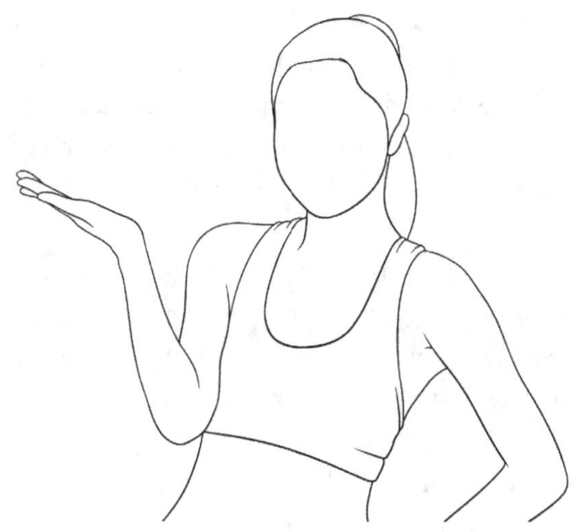

As the EmpowerFit 30-Day Fitness Challenge nears its conclusion, remember that your journey toward strength, confidence, and well-being extends far beyond these 30 days. Embrace this time as the beginning of a lifelong commitment to prioritizing self-care and adopting healthy habits. Your health and happiness deserve consistent attention and nurturing, and you hold the power to make lasting positive changes in your life. Here's why you should continue prioritizing self-care and adopting healthy habits beyond the challenge:

1. **Sustaining Progress:** The 30-day challenge has likely shown you the incredible potential you possess to transform physically and mentally. By continuing to prioritize self-care, you sustain and build upon the progress you've achieved during the challenge.

2. **Long-Term Health Benefits:** Investing in self-care and healthy habits yields significant long-term health benefits. Regular exercise, balanced nutrition, and mindfulness positively impact your physical well-being, mental clarity, and emotional resilience.

3. **Increased Energy and Vitality:** Self-care practices infuse your life with energy and vitality. When you take care of yourself, you feel more alive, motivated, and capable of tackling life's challenges with enthusiasm.

4. **Stress Management:** Self-care techniques, such as exercise, meditation, or spending time in nature, help you manage stress effectively. They empower you to navigate daily stressors with

grace and maintain a sense of inner peace.

5. Enhanced Self-Confidence: Adopting healthy habits and prioritizing self-care contribute to enhanced self-confidence and a positive self-image. Embrace the strength and capabilities you've discovered during the challenge, and let them empower you in all areas of life.

6. Setting an Example: By prioritizing self-care and healthy habits, you set a powerful example for others—family, friends, and loved ones. Your commitment inspires and motivates them to embark on their wellness journeys.

7. Lifelong Learning and Growth: Self-care is an ongoing journey of learning and growth. As you explore different practices and adapt them to suit your needs, you cultivate a deeper understanding of yourself and your capabilities.

8. Mind-Body Connection: Embrace the mind-body connection you've experienced during the challenge, as it enables you to better understand how your physical and mental well-being are intertwined. Nurturing this connection enriches your overall quality of life.

9. Joy and Fulfillment: Prioritizing self-care allows you to find joy and fulfillment in the little moments of everyday life. It empowers you to embrace self-compassion, celebrate progress, and find beauty in your journey.

10. Empowerment and Resilience: Embrace the knowledge that prioritizing self-care and adopting healthy habits is an empowering act of self-love. It equips you with resilience and strength to face any obstacles that come your way.

The EmpowerFit 30-day challenge is just the beginning—a catalyst for lifelong transformation. Embrace the profound impact of self-care and healthy habits on your well-being, relationships, and success in all areas of life. Continue to celebrate progress over perfection, be gentle with yourself, and take steps every day to nourish your body, mind, and soul. The EmpowerFit community stands with you, supporting and celebrating your journey every step of the way.

Let the end of the challenge be the beginning of a lifelong commitment to your health, happiness, and empowerment. With every choice you make to prioritize self-care, you fuel the fire of your strength, and you become a radiant force of positive change. Keep shining, EmpowerFit, and let your light illuminate the world around you!

The Mind–Body Connection

Mental and Physical Well-Being

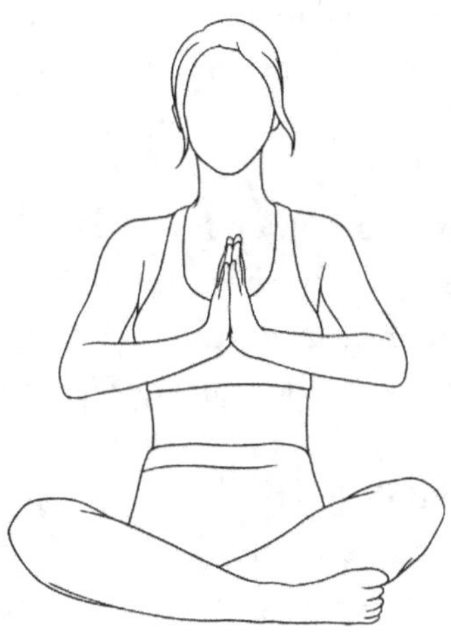

The relationship between mental health and physical well-being is profound and interconnected. Our minds and bodies are intricately linked, and taking care of one aspect positively impacts the other. Here's how mental health and physical well-being are interrelated and some strategies to maintain a positive body image:

Relationship Between Mental Health and Physical Well-being:

1. Stress and Cortisol: Mental stress can lead to the release of cortisol, a stress hormone, which, when consistently elevated, can negatively impact physical health, including immune function, metabolism, and cardiovascular health.

2. Mind-Body Connection: Our thoughts, emotions, and beliefs influence physical sensations and bodily functions. For instance, anxiety can lead to muscle tension, and chronic stress can manifest in physical symptoms like headaches or digestive issues.

3. Physical Activity and Mood: Engaging in regular physical activity, such as exercise, has been shown to release endorphins, the "feel-good" neurotransmitters, which can improve mood and reduce feelings of anxiety and depression.

4. Sleep and Mental Health: Quality sleep is vital for mental health and physical restoration. Poor sleep can negatively impact mood, cognitive function, and immune health.

5. Nutrition and Mental Clarity: Proper nutrition provides the brain with essential nutrients for optimal functioning. Balanced diets rich in vitamins, minerals, and healthy fats are associated with improved mental clarity and emotional stability.

Strategies to Maintain a Positive Body Image:

1. Practice Self-Compassion: Be kind and gentle with yourself. Recognize that everyone has unique physical traits, and focus on embracing and appreciating your body for what it enables you to do.

2. Limit Media Exposure: Be mindful of the media you consume. Reduce exposure to images that promote unrealistic beauty standards and instead seek out diverse representations of bodies.

3. Surround Yourself with Positive Influences: Build a supportive network of friends and loved ones who uplift and celebrate each other's bodies and accomplishments.

4. Focus on What Your Body Can Do: Shift the focus from appearance to function. Celebrate your body's strength, resilience, and capabilities, regardless of its shape or size.

5. Challenge Negative Thoughts: When negative thoughts about your body arise, challenge them with positive affirmations and realistic perspectives.

6. Set Realistic Goals: Focus on health-related goals rather than aesthetics. Set achievable and realistic goals that support your physical and mental well-being.

7. Engage in Physical Activities You Enjoy: Find physical activities that bring you joy and make you feel good about yourself. Move your body in ways that feel empowering and fulfilling.

8. Practice Mindfulness: Engage in mindfulness practices, such as meditation or deep breathing, to foster a greater sense of self-awareness and acceptance.

9. Avoid Comparison: Recognize that comparing yourself to others is unproductive and can harm your self-esteem. Your body is unique, and comparing it to others is an unfair comparison.

10. Seek Professional Support: If negative body image significantly impacts your mental health, consider seeking support from a therapist or counselor who specializes in body image issues and self-esteem.

Remember that your body is an incredible vessel that carries you through life's journey. It deserves to be treated with love, respect, and care. Embrace your body's uniqueness, celebrate its strengths, and prioritize self-compassion and self-care. By fostering a positive body image, you nurture both your mental and physical well-being, creating a harmonious and empowering relationship between mind and body.

Week 4: Rising Strong: Mind and Body Unite

Empowering Fusion Workouts

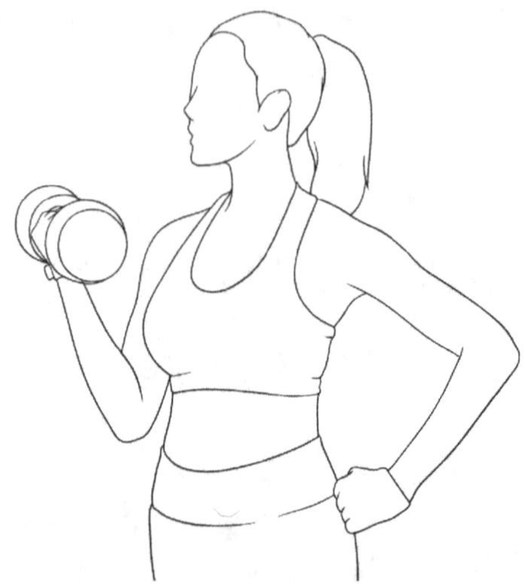

Congratulations on reaching this pinnacle of your EmpowerFit journey. In Week 4, we delve into the empowering world of Fusion Workouts—a harmonious blend of exercises that fuse the power of various disciplines to elevate your physical and mental prowess. These workouts embody the essence of our holistic approach to fitness, unifying the mind and body in a dynamic, invigorating synergy.

Fusion Workouts challenge your body in new ways, promoting functional strength, balance, and agility. They engage your mind with their creativity, keeping you fully present and immersed in the joy of movement. As you embrace these empowering sessions, you'll discover that the whole truly is greater than the sum of its parts.

Get ready to unlock your potential and rise strong with

Fusion Workouts that infuse your journey with vibrancy and excitement. Here are some example workouts to fuel your inspiration:

1. **Yoga HIIT Fusion:** A fusion of high-intensity interval training (HIIT) and yoga, this workout combines cardiovascular bursts with flowing yoga sequences. Experience the energizing rhythm of HIIT with moments of mindful grounding, leaving you empowered and centered.

2. **Dance and Strength Fusion:** Groove to the beat as you blend dance-inspired movements with strength exercises. This workout celebrates self-expression and encourages you to find joy in the beauty of dance while building strength and endurance.

3. **Pilates and Barre Fusion:** Combine the core-strengthening benefits of Pilates with the grace and poise of barre workouts. Sculpt and lengthen your muscles, enhancing your posture and flexibility in a dynamic fusion.

4. **Kickboxing Yoga Fusion:** Unleash your inner warrior with a fusion of kickboxing and yoga. Channel your strength and resilience as you alternate between empowering punches and kicks, followed by grounding and restorative yoga poses.

5. **Aqua Zumba and Aqua Aerobics Fusion:** Take your workout to the pool with a fun combination of Aqua Zumba's lively dance routines and Aqua Aerobics' low-impact cardio movements. Feel weightless as you boost your heart rate and embrace the refreshing aquatic environment.

Each Fusion Workout presents an opportunity for self-discovery and growth as you embrace the interplay between mind and body. Feel the empowerment that arises when you push boundaries and explore the synergy of different exercise disciplines.

Week 4 invites you to dance with your strength, grace, and newfound confidence. Embrace the exhilaration of Fusion Workouts as you rise strong and united—mind and body harmonizing in a celebration of your empowered spirit.

Let the empowering rhythm of Fusion Workouts propel you forward as you conclude this transformative journey. Your commitment, determination, and growth have ignited a spark within you that will continue to blaze brightly beyond these 30 days.

Keep thriving, keep embracing progress, and let your EmpowerFit journey be a testament to the extraordinary woman you are!

EmpowerFit Transformations

Inspiring Success Stories

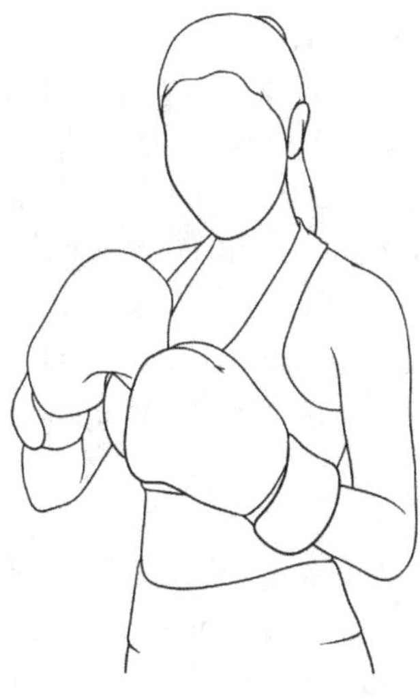

Here are some inspiring success stories from women who have completed the EmpowerFit 30-Day Fitness Challenge:

1. Sarah's Strength Journey: Sarah, a working mother of two, joined the EmpowerFit challenge to reclaim her physical and mental well-being. Through consistent dedication to the workouts and self-care practices, she witnessed incredible progress. Sarah's strength increased significantly, allowing her to lift weights she never thought possible. Moreover, her positive body image and self-confidence skyrocketed, inspiring her to take on new challenges in her personal and professional life. Sarah now embraces her role as a strong, empowered woman and continues to prioritize her health and well-being.

2. Lily's Mind-Body Connection: Lily, a college student struggling with stress and anxiety, found solace in the EmpowerFit challenge. The combination of yoga, Pilates, and mindfulness techniques allowed her to strengthen the mind-body connection. As she progressed through the challenge, Lily experienced reduced anxiety and a sense of calmness. She found that practicing self-compassion during workouts translated into her daily life, transforming her relationship with herself and others. Lily now carries the tools she learned in the challenge to manage stress and embrace a more mindful, balanced lifestyle.

3. Emily's Transformation: Emily, a passionate dancer, and performer, joined the EmpowerFit challenge to improve her overall fitness and stamina. Throughout the 30 days, she witnessed her body becoming leaner and stronger, allowing her to execute complex dance moves with greater ease. More importantly, the challenge empowered Emily to embrace her body's uniqueness, fostering a deep sense of body appreciation. With newfound confidence, Emily now takes the stage with radiant energy, inspiring others to embrace their passions fearlessly.

4. Alex's Empowerment Journey: Alex, a mother of three and a survivor of a personal life challenge, embarked on the EmpowerFit challenge to rebuild her strength and reclaim her sense of self. Over the 30 days, Alex found a supportive community that uplifted and encouraged her every step of the way. The empowering exercises and motivational content inspired Alex to set new personal and fitness goals. Today, she is not only a stronger and fitter version of herself but also an advocate for empowering women to prioritize self-care and resilience.

5. Samantha's Wellness Revelation: Samantha, a busy professional, joined the EmpowerFit challenge with a desire to improve her overall well-being. Through the diverse workouts and self-care practices, she discovered the joy of movement and the importance of taking time for herself. Samantha now prioritizes daily walks, meditation, and nutritious meals to maintain her newfound balance and vitality. The challenge ignited a passion for fitness and self-discovery, inspiring Samantha to embrace a holistic approach to wellness in her life.

These success stories showcase the transformative power of the EmpowerFit 30-Day Fitness Challenge. Through dedication, support, and a commitment to self-improvement, these women have embraced their strength, resilience, and inner power. Their stories serve as an inspiration to all women embarking on their fitness journeys, empowering them to prioritize self-care, embrace progress, and believe in their potential to achieve remarkable transformations. Keep shining, EmpowerFit, and let your journey be a beacon of inspiration for others seeking to embrace their empowerment and well-being!

Nourishing Your Empowerment

Balanced Meal Plans

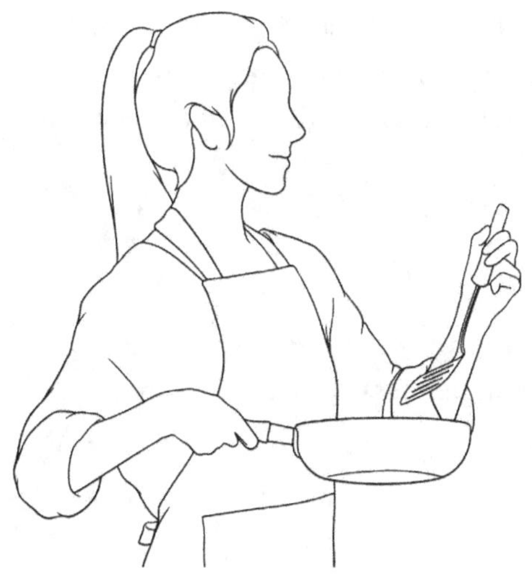

Here are some sample meal plans and healthy recipes that align with balanced eating for optimal performance:

Sample Meal Plan 1:

Breakfast:

- **Veggie Omelette:** Whisk together 2 eggs with diced bell peppers, spinach, and tomatoes. Cook in a non-stick pan with a little olive oil until set. Serve with whole-grain toast and a side of fresh fruit.

Lunch:

- **Grilled Chicken Salad:** Grilled chicken breast served on a bed of mixed greens, cherry tomatoes, cucumbers, and avocado slices. Dress with a light vinaigrette dressing.

Snack:

- **Greek Yogurt with Berries:** Top a cup of Greek yogurt with fresh berries, a drizzle of honey, and a sprinkle of granola.

Dinner:

- **Baked Salmon with Quinoa and Roasted Vegetables:** Season salmon fillet with herbs and bake in the oven. Serve with cooked quinoa and a mix of roasted broccoli, carrots, and bell peppers.

Sample Meal Plan 2:

Breakfast:

- **Overnight Oats:** Combine rolled oats with almond milk, chia seeds, and your choice of nuts and fruits. Let it sit in the fridge overnight, and enjoy a ready-to-eat breakfast in the morning.

Lunch:

- **Turkey and Hummus Wrap:** Fill a whole-grain wrap with lean turkey slices, hummus, sliced cucumbers, tomatoes, and lettuce.

Snack:

- **Veggie Sticks with Hummus:** Enjoy carrot, cucumber, and bell pepper sticks with a side of hummus for dipping.

Dinner:

- **Stir-Fried Tofu with Brown Rice and Broccoli:** Stir-fry tofu with garlic, ginger, and your favorite veggies. Serve over cooked brown rice.

Sample Meal Plan 3:

Breakfast:

- Berry Chia Pudding: Combine chia seeds with almond milk and a handful of mixed berries. Let it sit overnight in the fridge and enjoy a creamy, nutritious breakfast.

Lunch:

- Quinoa Avocado Salad: Mix cooked quinoa with avocado slices, cherry tomatoes, cucumber, red onion, and fresh cilantro. Dress with a squeeze of lime juice and a drizzle of olive oil.

Snack:

- Apple Slices with Almond Butter: Dip crisp apple slices in almond butter for a satisfying and energizing snack.

Dinner:

- Spicy Chickpea Stew: Sauté onions, garlic, and diced bell peppers. Add canned chickpeas, diced tomatoes, vegetable broth, and a blend of spices like cumin, paprika, and cayenne pepper. Simmer until the flavors meld into a hearty stew.

Sample Meal Plan 4:

Breakfast:

- Greek Yogurt Parfait: Layer Greek yogurt with granola, sliced bananas, and a drizzle of honey for a protein-rich breakfast.

Lunch:

- Lentil and Vegetable Stir-Fry: Sauté bell peppers, broccoli, and snap peas. Add cooked lentils and a splash of soy sauce for a nutritious and flavorful lunch.

Snack:

- Hummus and Veggie Stuffed Pita: Fill a whole-wheat pita with hummus, sliced cucumbers, cherry tomatoes, and baby spinach.

Dinner:

- Grilled Portobello Mushroom Burger: Marinate portobello mushroom caps in balsamic vinegar and grill until tender. Serve on a whole-grain bun with lettuce, tomato, and a dollop of avocado spread.

Sample Meal Plan 5:

Breakfast:

- Mediterranean Omelette: Whisk together 2 eggs with diced red bell peppers, spinach, black olives, and feta cheese. Cook in a non-stick pan until set.

Lunch:

- Quinoa Tabouli Salad: Mix cooked quinoa with chopped cucumber, cherry tomatoes, fresh parsley, mint, and a lemon-olive oil dressing.

Snack:

- Greek Yogurt with Pistachios: Top Greek yogurt with crushed pistachios and a sprinkle of cinnamon.

Dinner:

- Lemon Herb Grilled Chicken: Marinate chicken breasts in a mixture of lemon juice, olive oil, garlic, and a blend of herbs. Grill until cooked through, and serve with roasted vegetables.

Sample Meal Plan 6:

- Avocado Toast: Spread mashed avocado on whole-grain toast and top with sliced radishes and a sprinkle of black sesame seeds.

Lunch:

- Greek Chickpea Salad: Combine canned chickpeas with diced cucumber, cherry tomatoes, red onion, kalamata olives, and crumbled feta cheese. Dress with a lemon-oregano vinaigrette.

Snack:

- Carrot and Cucumber Sticks with Tzatziki: Dip carrot and cucumber sticks in tzatziki sauce for a refreshing and satisfying snack.

Dinner:

- Baked Cod with Mediterranean Salsa: Season cod fillets with lemon zest, garlic, and dried oregano. Bake until flaky, and serve with a fresh salsa made from diced tomatoes, red onion, capers, and fresh basil.

Sample Meal Plan 7:

Breakfast:

- Smoothie Bowl: Blend frozen mixed berries, banana, spinach, and a scoop of plant-based protein powder. Top with sliced kiwi, coconut flakes, and chia seeds.

Lunch:

- Tofu and Veggie Stir-Fry: Sauté tofu cubes with bell

peppers, broccoli, and snow peas. Toss with a savory soy-ginger sauce and serve over brown rice.

Snack:

- Rice Cakes with Almond Butter and Berries: Spread almond butter on rice cakes and top with fresh berries.

Dinner:

- Lentil Curry: Simmer cooked lentils with coconut milk, diced tomatoes, and a blend of curry spices. Serve over cauliflower rice for a nourishing and flavorful dinner.

These diverse and nutritious meal plans will support your EmpowerFit journey with a variety of delicious, wholesome foods. Feel free to adjust portion sizes and ingredients according to your preferences and dietary needs. Embrace the nourishing power of these meals and continue to thrive with strength and grace!

Healthy Recipes

1. Snack: Quinoa Stuffed Bell Peppers:

- Cut the tops off bell peppers and remove the seeds. Precook quinoa with vegetable broth. In a pan, sauté onions, garlic, and your choice of diced vegetables. Mix the sautéed veggies with the cooked quinoa and stuff the bell peppers. Bake in the oven until the peppers are tender.

2. Dinner: Chickpea and Vegetable Curry:

- In a pot, sauté onions, garlic, and ginger. Add curry powder, turmeric, cumin, and paprika. Add diced tomatoes, vegetable broth, and canned chickpeas. Simmer until the flavors meld and the sauce thickens. Serve over brown rice with a side of steamed broccoli.

3. Lunch: Mango Avocado Salad:

- Toss diced mango, avocado, cherry tomatoes, red onions, and cilantro in a bowl. Dress with lime juice, a drizzle of olive oil, and a pinch of salt.

4. Breakfast: Blueberry Almond Overnight Oats

- Mix rolled oats, almond milk, chia seeds, a handful of blueberries, and a drizzle of honey in a jar. Refrigerate overnight and enjoy a nutritious and filling breakfast.

5. Lunch: Grilled Vegetable Quinoa Bowl

- Grill an assortment of colorful vegetables (zucchini, bell peppers, eggplant) and toss with cooked quinoa. Top with crumbled feta cheese and a lemon-herb dressing.

6. Snack: Energy-Boosting Trail Mix

- Combine roasted almonds, walnuts, pumpkin seeds, dried cranberries, and dark chocolate chips for a satisfying and portable snack.

7. Dinner: Baked Salmon with Asparagus and Lemon

- Place salmon fillets on a baking sheet with asparagus spears. Drizzle with olive oil, lemon juice, and garlic. Bake until salmon is flaky and asparagus is tender.

8. Dessert: Dark Chocolate Avocado Mousse

- Blend ripe avocado, unsweetened cocoa powder, a splash of almond milk, and a touch of honey until smooth and creamy. Chill in the refrigerator for a luscious and guilt-free dessert.

9. Breakfast: Banana Nut Smoothie

- Blend frozen bananas, almond milk, a spoonful of almond butter, and a sprinkle of cinnamon for a creamy and nutritious breakfast smoothie.

10. Lunch: Caprese Stuffed Avocado

- Scoop out the flesh of halved avocados and fill with cherry tomatoes, fresh mozzarella balls, and basil leaves. Drizzle with balsamic glaze.

11. Snack: Greek Yogurt Parfait with Berries

- Layer Greek yogurt with mixed berries, granola, and a drizzle of honey for a protein-packed and refreshing snack.

12. Dinner: Turkey and Vegetable Stir-Fry

- Sauté ground turkey with a mix of colorful vegetables (bell peppers, carrots, snap peas) and a savory stir-fry sauce. Serve over brown rice.

13. Dessert: Berry Chia Seed Popsicles

- Blend mixed berries, almond milk, chia seeds, and a touch of honey. Pour the mixture into popsicle molds and freeze for a refreshing and nutritious treat.

Enjoy the delightful flavors and nourishing ingredients of these healthy recipes, and let them complement your EmpowerFit journey with vibrant and balanced meals. Bon appétit!

Remember to adjust portion sizes according to your individual calorie needs and activity levels. These meal plans and recipes offer a balanced combination of macronutrients and essential nutrients to fuel your body and support optimal performance. Prioritize whole, unprocessed foods, and listen to your body's hunger and fullness cues. Enjoy the process of exploring new flavors and nourishing yourself with wholesome, delicious meals!

Setting New Horizons

Beyond the 30-Day Challenge

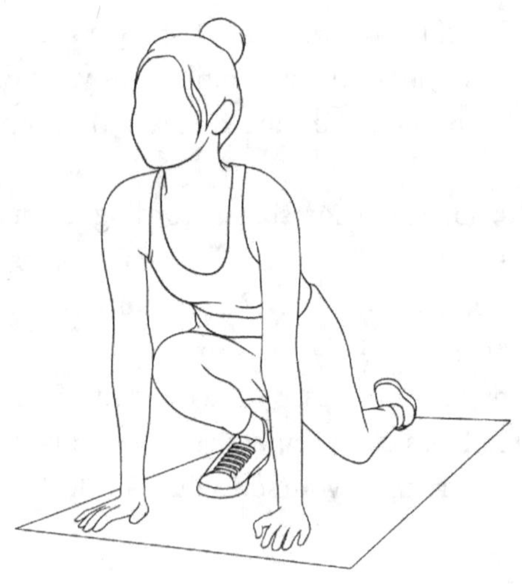

Setting new fitness goals beyond the 30-day challenge is an exciting and empowering step in your journey toward a healthy lifestyle. Here's a guide to help you set meaningful goals and maintain a balanced and sustainable approach to your well-being:

1. **Reflect on Your Journey:** Take some time to reflect on your experiences during the 30-day challenge. Celebrate the progress you've made, the obstacles you've overcome, and the lessons you've learned. Use this reflection to gain insights into your strengths, areas for improvement, and what motivates you to keep going.

2. **Define Specific and Realistic Goals:** Set specific and achievable fitness goals that align with your aspirations. Whether it's improving your strength, running a certain distance, or mastering a particular yoga pose, make sure your goals are attainable within a reasonable timeframe.

3. **Create a Plan:** Break down your goals into smaller milestones and create a plan to achieve them. Design a workout routine that incorporates a mix of cardiovascular exercises, strength training, flexibility, and mindfulness practices. Include rest days and recovery to prevent burnout and support overall well-being.

4. **Stay Flexible:** Life is full of unpredictability, and it's essential to stay flexible with your goals. If circumstances change or setbacks occur, be kind to yourself and adjust your plan as needed. Remember, progress is not always linear, and setbacks are growth opportunities.

5. Find Enjoyment: Explore various physical activities and exercises to find what brings you joy and fulfillment. When you enjoy your workouts, they become sustainable habits rather than chores. Embrace activities that make you feel strong, confident, and alive.

6. Seek Support and Accountability: Share your goals with friends, family, or fitness buddies who can offer encouragement and support. Join fitness classes, groups, or online communities that align with your interests to stay motivated and accountable.

7. Prioritize Self-Care: A healthy lifestyle encompasses more than just physical fitness. Prioritize self-care through sufficient sleep, stress management techniques, and nourishing foods. Engage in activities that promote mental well-being and balance in your life.

8. Embrace Progress Over Perfection: Remember that progress is a journey, and it's okay to have ups and downs. Embrace every step of progress, no matter how small, and celebrate your achievements. Focus on the positive changes you've made and the improvements in your overall well-being.

9. Stay Curious and Open-Minded: Be curious about your body's capabilities and open to trying new activities or workouts. Variety keeps fitness enjoyable and prevents monotony.

10. Practice Self-Compassion: Be patient and compassionate with yourself. Acknowledge that fitness and lifestyle changes take time and effort. Celebrate the process, honor your body, and be proud of every step you take towards a healthier, happier you.

Setting new fitness goals and maintaining a healthy lifestyle is a testament to your commitment to self-improvement and well-being. Your journey is unique, and each day presents new growth opportunities. Embrace the empowering transformation you've initiated and carry it with you beyond the 30-day challenge. Continue to be the strong, resilient, and empowered woman you are, and let your journey inspire others to embrace their strength and vitality. With every choice you make toward your well-being, you pave the way for a life filled with energy, joy, and self-empowerment. Keep shining and thriving, EmpowerFit!

Conclusion

Carrying the EmpowerFit Spirit

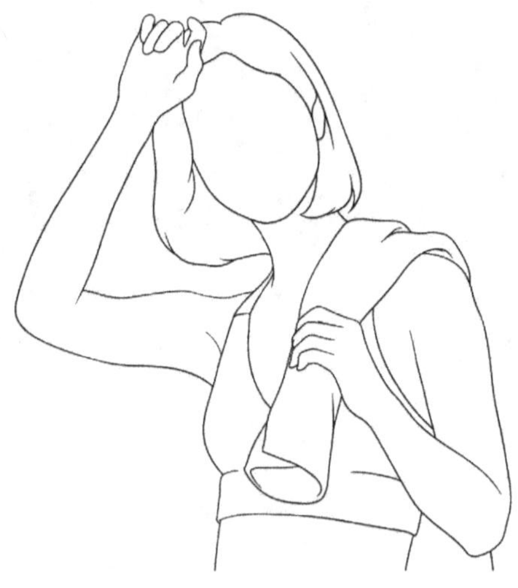

As we conclude this book, take a moment to reflect on the incredible journey you've embarked on—the EmpowerFit journey towards strength, confidence, and well-being. Throughout these pages, you've explored diverse workouts, embraced self-care, and delved into the profound connection between your mind and body. You've witnessed your body's capabilities, your resilience, and your growth potential. You've discovered the beauty of progress over perfection and the power of self-compassion. As you close this chapter, remember that your journey doesn't end here—it's just the beginning of an empowering, lifelong transformation.

In your hands lies a story of determination, perseverance, and self-discovery. You are a testament to the strength that resides within you—a strength that extends far beyond physical prowess. You've learned that your well-being encompasses more than just your body; it's a harmony of body, mind, and soul. Embrace the profound impact of self-care and healthy habits on your physical and mental well-being. Embrace the joy of movement, the beauty of self-acceptance, and the empowering process of progress.

As you venture beyond the 30-day challenge, remember to celebrate every step of progress you make—no matter how big or small. Your journey may present challenges and setbacks, but these are opportunities for growth and resilience. Be kind to yourself and practice self-compassion, for you are a work in progress, continuously evolving and blossoming into the empowered woman you're destined to be.

Your EmpowerFit journey is not just about achieving specific goals; it's about nurturing yourself—mind, body, and soul. Embrace self-care as an act of self-love, and let it guide you towards a balanced and fulfilling life. Remember that every day is a chance to make choices that empower you and contribute to your well-being. Surround yourself with supportive and uplifting influences, and let your light shine brightly, illuminating the world around you.

In closing, I invite you to celebrate your progress and growth. Celebrate every time you step out of your comfort zone, every time you choose nourishing foods, and every time you embrace mindfulness and self-awareness. Celebrate the vibrant, empowered woman you've become and the endless possibilities that lie ahead.

As you continue your journey, let the fire of empowerment burn brightly within you. Take the strength and wisdom you've gained and share it with others, inspiring them to embark on their paths of self-discovery and well-being.

Thank you for being a part of the EmpowerFit community. You are not alone in your journey; you are supported and celebrated by a community of strong, resilient, and empowered women. Embrace the power within you, keep thriving, and let your journey be a beacon of inspiration for those around you.

Maintaining a Healthy Lifestyle

Continuing the EmpowerFit Legacy

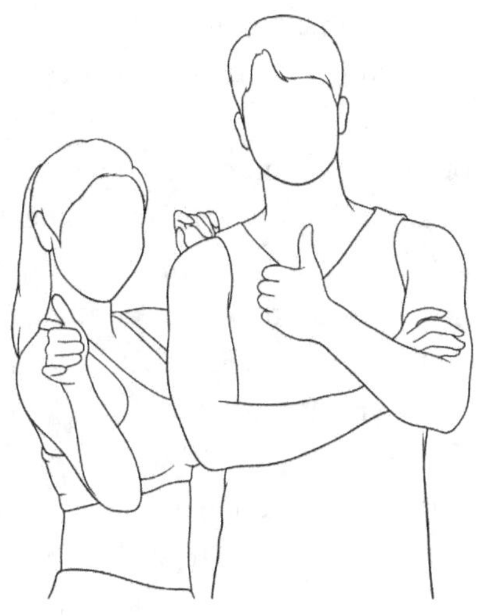

As you stand at the crossroads of the EmpowerFit journey, let the flame of newfound confidence and strength burn brightly within you. You've embraced the power that resides within your mind, body, and soul, and now it's time to carry that fire with you as you continue your fitness journey.

With each step you take, know that you are capable of achieving remarkable transformations. Your journey is unique, and every milestone, every challenge, and every triumph is a testament to your strength and determination. Embrace the joy of progress and the beauty of self-discovery.

Remember that your journey is not just about reaching a destination; it's about the growth, empowerment, and resilience you cultivate along the way. You've witnessed the power of self-care, the importance of balance, and the impact of a positive mindset. These invaluable lessons will serve as your guiding light as you navigate life's twists and turns.

In moments of doubt, remember the woman you've become—the woman who radiates confidence, embraces her uniqueness, and lifts others with her empowered spirit. Embrace the imperfections, the setbacks, and the uncertainties, for they are part of the journey that shapes you into the empowered woman you are meant to be.

Surround yourself with like-minded individuals who uplift and support you, and never hesitate to seek inspiration from the EmpowerFit community. You are not alone; we walk this path together, empowering and celebrating each other's triumphs.

As you continue your fitness journey, know that the strength you've discovered transcends the physical. Your strength resides in your unwavering determination, your commitment to growth, and your ability to rise above challenges with grace and resilience.

Your journey is a testament to your power, your worth, and your endless potential. Embrace every opportunity to nourish your mind, body, and soul, and let the flame of confidence and strength guide you to new heights.

Keep shining, keep thriving, and keep empowering yourself and others. Your journey is boundless, and the world awaits the brilliance you bring to it. With every step, you leave a trail of inspiration and empowerment for generations to come.

You are strong, you are capable, and you are enough. Carry the EmpowerFit spirit with you always, and let your fitness journey be a testimony to the extraordinary woman you are.

With an unwavering belief in your power,

EmpowerFit Community

30-DAY CHALLENGE

This comprehensive day-by-day guide offers sample workouts and exercises, providing you with the option to follow a structured plan. However, remember that this cheat sheet is a flexible resource, and you can tailor it to suit your preferences and fitness level. Whether you choose to follow the daily challenges or design your personalized routine, the EmpowerFit Cheat Sheet is here to support your continued journey of empowerment and well-being. Embrace this empowering tool, celebrate your progress, and remember that you have the strength and grace to rise strong, both within and beyond these pages.

Week 1: Building Strength and Resilience
  Day 1:

- Warm-up: Dynamic stretches (arm circles, leg swings, high knees)
- Foundation-Building Exercises: Bodyweight squats, push-

ups, plank variations
- Cardiovascular Endurance Workout: 20 minutes of brisk walking or jogging

Day 2:

- Warm-up: Jumping jacks, hip circles, shoulder rolls
- Cardiovascular Endurance Workout: 30 minutes of cycling or stationary biking

Day 3:

- Warm-up: Standing side lunges, arm crosses, neck rolls
- Strength Training for Beginners: Dumbbell curls, tricep dips, lunges with dumbbell press

Day 4:

- Rest Day: Focus on self-care and relaxation

Day 5:

- Warm-up: Jump rope, leg swings, arm circles
- Cardiovascular Endurance Workout: 20 minutes of high-intensity interval training (HIIT) with jumping jacks, burpees, and mountain climbers

Day 6:

- Warm-up: Hip hinges, torso twists, ankle circles
- Cardiovascular Endurance Workout: 30 minutes of swim-

ming or water aerobics

Day 7:

- Warm-up: Cat-cow stretches, neck stretches, wrist circles
- Strength Training for Beginners: Bodyweight lunges, assisted push-ups, seated dumbbell shoulder press

Week 2: Empowering with Cardio and Strength
  Day 8:

- Warm-up: Arm circles, leg swings, knee hugs
- Cardiovascular and Strength Workout Combined: Circuit training with jumping squats, push-ups, and mountain climbers

Day 9:

- Warm-up: Jumping jacks, high knees, shoulder circles
- Cardiovascular and Strength Workout Combined: Dance-inspired cardio with squats and arm movements

Day 10:

- Warm-up: Torso twists, hip circles, ankle rolls
- Cardiovascular and Strength Workout Combined: Barre exercises with pliés, leg lifts, and arm toning movements

Day 11:

- Rest Day: Focus on rest and rejuvenation

Day 12:

- Warm-up: Jump rope, side lunges, arm swings
- Cardiovascular and Strength Workout Combined: Kickboxing moves with lunges, punches, and front kicks

Day 13:

- Warm-up: Wrist circles, neck stretches, hip hinges
- Cardiovascular and Strength Workout Combined: Aqua Zumba with salsa-inspired moves in the pool

Day 14:

- Warm-up: Cat-cow stretches, shoulder rolls, ankle circles
- Cardiovascular and Strength Workout Combined: Pilates-inspired exercises with leg lifts and core work

Week 3: Finding Balance with Yoga and Pilates
Day 15:

- Warm-up: Sun salutations, neck rolls, ankle stretches
- Yoga and Pilates Fusion: Flowing yoga sequence with Pilates core exercises

Day 16:

- Warm-up: Shoulder rolls, wrist circles, torso twists
- Yoga and Pilates Fusion: Yoga poses with Pilates leg and arm movements

Day 17:

- Warm-up: Ankle circles, hip hinges, standing side stretches
- Yoga and Pilates Fusion: Balancing yoga poses with Pilates back exercises

Day 18:

- Rest Day: Focus on self-care and relaxation

Day 19:

- Warm-up: Arm swings, leg swings, knee hugs
- Yoga and Pilates Fusion: Yoga stretches with Pilates side body and oblique exercises

Day 20:

- Warm-up: Shoulder circles, hip circles, wrist stretches
- Yoga and Pilates Fusion: Flowing yoga sequence with Pilates roll-ups and teasers

Day 21:

- Warm-up: Neck stretches, ankle stretches, torso twists
- Yoga and Pilates Fusion: Yoga poses with Pilates spine stretches

Week 4: Rising Strong: Mind and Body Unite
Day 22:

- Warm-up: Jumping jacks, high knees, arm crosses
- Empowering Fusion Workout: Yoga HIIT Fusion with cardiovascular bursts and yoga flows

Day 23:

- Warm-up: Leg swings, arm circles, ankle rolls
- Empowering Fusion Workout: Dance and Strength Fusion with dance-inspired cardio and strength exercises

Day 24:

- Warm-up: Hip circles, shoulder rolls, wrist circles
- Empowering Fusion Workout: Pilates and Barre Fusion with core work and graceful barre movements

Day 25:

- Rest Day: Focus on rest and rejuvenation

Day 26:

- Warm-up: Jump rope, torso twists, leg swings
- Empowering Fusion Workout: Kickboxing Yoga Fusion with energizing kickboxing and grounding yoga

Day 27:

- Warm-up: Wrist circles, shoulder rolls, neck stretches
- Empowering Fusion Workout: Aqua Zumba and Aqua Aerobics Fusion with water-based cardio and dance

Day 28:

- Warm-up: Cat-cow stretches, hip hinges, arm circles
- Empowering Fusion Workout: Fusion of Yoga and HIIT with dynamic yoga poses and high-intensity intervals

Week 5: Embracing Progress and Beyond
Day 29:

- Warm-up: Standing side stretches, hip circles, ankle stretches
- Empowering Fusion Workout: Final Fusion Challenge—Combine elements from previous Fusion Workouts for a creative and invigorating session

Day 30:

- Warm-up: Full-body stretches, deep breathing
- Reflection and Celebration: Take time to reflect on your EmpowerFit journey, celebrate your progress, and set new goals for continued growth.

Congratulations on completing the EmpowerFit 30-day challenge! May this cheat sheet inspire you to thrive with strength and grace, embracing the empowerment that lies within you.

Afterthoughts

As we come to the end of this transformative journey in EmpowerFit, I want to take a moment to express my heartfelt gratitude for being a part of this empowering community. Your dedication to self-improvement, your commitment to growth, and your unwavering spirit have made this journey all the more rewarding.

If you've found inspiration, motivation, and empowerment within the pages of EmpowerFit, I kindly ask you to consider leaving a review for this book. Your honest feedback will help others discover the empowering world of EmpowerFit and embark on their journeys toward strength and grace.

Moreover, I encourage you to share this book with your friends and family. You have experienced the transformative power of Fusion Workouts, the beauty of self-care, and the importance of embracing progress. By recommending this book, you gift them the keys to unlocking their potential and embracing a balanced, vibrant lifestyle.

As you continue your journey beyond these pages, remember that you are part of a supportive community of strong, empowered women. Share your triumphs, challenges, and empowering moments with us, and let us continue uplifting each other in our pursuit of well-being and self-discovery.

Your journey is far from over—it's just the beginning of a life filled with vitality, strength, and empowerment. Let your light shine brightly, and let your empowerment be a beacon of inspiration for others.

Thank you for being a part of EmpowerFit and for joining me in this empowering adventure. With each step, we grow stronger together.

With gratitude and anticipation for the impact of EmpowerFit in your life,

Aria Evergreen